THE ULTIMATE LOCUM DOCTOR GUIDE

UniAdmissions

ISBN: 978-1-915091-28-4

Published by *RAR Medical Services Limited*

www.uniadmissions.co.uk

info@uniadmissions.co.uk

Tel: 0208 068 0438

THE ULTIMATE LOCUM DOCTOR GUIDE

DR MOJI AKINSOLA

DR ANIL AGARWAL

DR RANJNA GARG

EDITOR: DR ROHAN AGARWAL

UniAdmissions

About the Authors

Dr Moji Akinsola

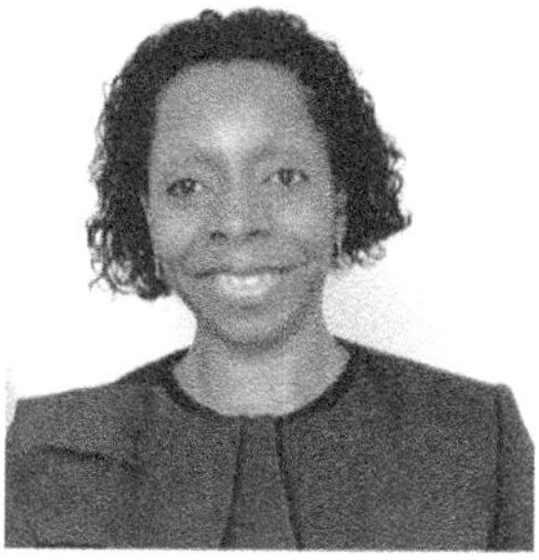

Dr Akinsola has been working as an NHS consultant since 2002. Her consultant career first started in Leicester and in 2004 she moved to Berkshire to work at the Wexham Park Hospital. It was here that she took the challenge of leading the service and training programme and became director for speciality training in the Thames Valley. Dr Akinsola has also coached, mentored, and supported trainees in difficulty. In 2016, she started locum work to provide herself with a better work-life balance. Her interests outside of work include listening to music, watching films, enjoying wildlife, and travelling.

Dr Anil K Agarwal

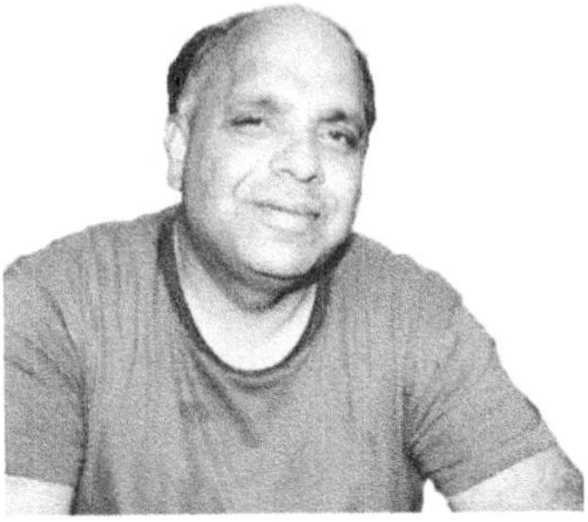

Dr Agarwal has over 35 years of experience in clinical teaching and research. For the last decade, he has been the lead of the Stroke Unit at Basildon University Hospital. Dr Agarwal has authored many publications in peer reviewed journals and authored "The Medical Consultant Interview book" and is also an MRCP (UK) PACES examiner. He is passionate about teaching and has taught hundreds of junior doctors and medical students. In his spare time, Dr Agarwal enjoys gardening, wildlife, and hiking.

Dr Ranjna Garg

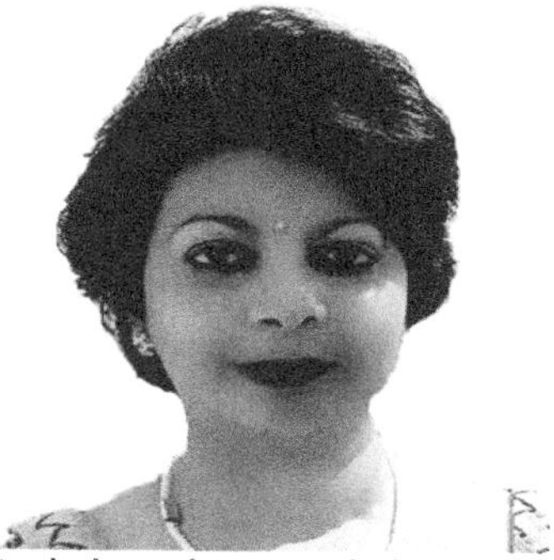

Dr Garg has been an NHS consultant since 2008. She is a consultant endocrinologist, diabetologist and a general physician. Her consultant career began in the Midlands and since has worked in several prestigious hospitals including the Royal Free Hospital in London, University Hospital London and London North West University Healthcare NHS Trust.

Dr Garg has prepared hundreds of junior doctors for postgraduate examinations and job interviews, a role she thoroughly enjoys. Additionally, Dr Garg has interviewed for London based medical schools. As well as her clinical work, Dr Garg has done significant research on the use of high strength insulin in patients with severe insulin resistance. In her spare time, Dr Garg enjoys running, photography and making candles.

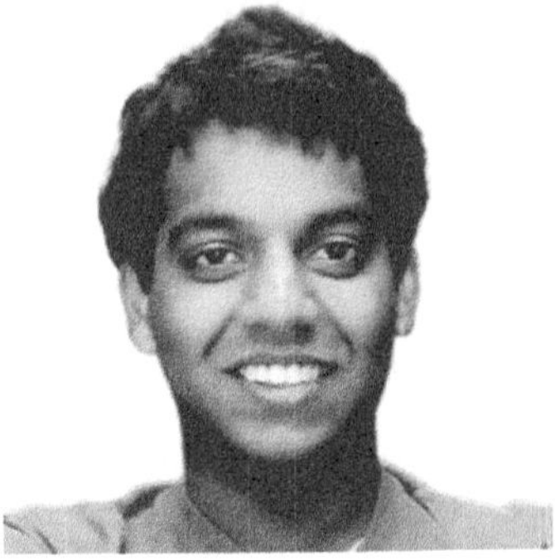

Dr Agarwal is the **Managing Director** at UniAdmissions and is responsible for its leadership and strategy. Rohan graduated from Gonville and Caius College, Cambridge and is a qualified doctor. He has tutored hundreds of successful Oxbridge and medical applicants. He has also authored numerous books on admissions tests and interviews. Rohan has taught physiology to undergraduates and interviewed medical school applicants for Cambridge. He has published research on bone physiology and writes education articles for The Independent, The Guardian and HuffPost. In his spare time, Rohan enjoys playing the piano and table tennis.

Preface

Congratulations on taking the first step in preparing to be a locum doctor. Being a locum has both its advantages and disadvantages, which you need to be aware of before starting this journey. It is important to be aware of the key differences between being a substantive and a locum doctor. Locum work is undertaken for many reasons but in all cases attention to detail is crucial. This book describes "life as a locum" and we will cover several aspects of locum life and provide helpful tips for doctors considering locum work. Although locum work is done at every level within the health sector, this book will focus on locum work conducted in a hospital and not in a GP practice.

We would like to thank Dr Archana Dhere (consultant physician) who shared her own experiences with us during the preparation of this book.

I hope you enjoy the book. As always, please let us know your thoughts and suggestions on what should be included in subsequent editions.

Dr Ranjna Garg

CONTENTS

List of tables

BASICS

WHAT IS A LOCUM DOCTOR?

The word locum comes from the Latin "locum tenens", which means, "place holder". A locum is a person who temporarily fulfils the duties of another. The General Medical Council (GMC) states, "a doctor in locum tenens is one who is standing in for an absent doctor, or temporarily covering a vacancy in an established post or position." A locum may refer to a doctor who is placed by a locum agency, GP chambers or a locum bank to work in a health care organisation or directly engage with a health care organisation or GP practise to provide short-term work.

Whilst the number of licensed doctors has remained relatively steady the number of doctors working in a locum capacity has increased from 13-18% in the years 2013 and 2017. In 2018, a report published by the GMC reported there were 12,000 more doctors undertaking locum work in the years 2013-2017 than in previous years. This is equivalent to 1 in 5 doctors.

Over the years, a shortage of NHS doctors has led to an increased demand for locum doctors. A recent British Medical Association (BMA) report estimated the number of NHS medical vacancies to be around 6634. The locum role has expanded to cover holidays as well as periods of sickness, maternity leave and gaps in rotas. Additionally, locums can be hired to fill positions that have not yet been filled. Three of the main medical areas experiencing shortages are emergency medicine, general practice and psychiatry. A survey of over 6000 foundation year 2 doctors found that in 2018, 37.7% immediately took up a specialty training post compared to 42.6% the year before. In addition, an increasing number of senior doctors are taking early retirement; the number of GPs claiming early NHS pension voluntarily increased from 198 in 2007 to 721 in 2017. All these factors have contributed to chronic staff shortages, highlighting the importance of locum doctors.

WHAT ARE THE DIFFERENCES BETWEEN A SUBSTANTIVE DOCTOR AND A LOCUM DOCTOR?

A permanent or a substantive doctor is a doctor who has an employment contract with an NHS trust, is a salaried GP or a partner in a GP practice. Usually this contract is permanent but can be of a fixed duration in the case of a trainee doctor. The doctor will be on the employee payroll, receive a monthly salary and will have pensionable earnings. They will also enjoy the benefits of being a permanent member of staff. On the other hand, a locum doctor is employed on a temporary basis and thus, does not receive the same benefits as a substantive doctor.

WHO ARE LOCUM DOCTORS?

A locum doctor can be full-time, part-time or occasional and be of any grade including trainee, GP, and consultant. GPs make up the highest percentage of locum doctors due to the nature of their work and many GPs prefer to do locum work instead of becoming a partner in a practice. Doctors will often take on short-term locum work while waiting for a permanent training position. There are some training locum positions that are referred to as locum appointment for training or LAT positions, which enable locum shifts to be undertaken to gain extra income while performing their primary job.

There is a growing trend of doctors who work as a locum for their first consultant job after receiving their Certificate of Completion Training (CCT); this allows them to gain crucial experience in the role before securing a permanent position. There is also a growing trend of consultants who have decided to do locum work. Thus, working as a locum is becoming increasingly popular in many grades of health care.

As a trainee doctor it is possible to take up a locum appointment for service (LAS), or locum appointment for training (LAT) post. For doctors in foundation years 1 and 2 these training posts may arise if vacancies have not been filled and are usually advertised locally. It is important to be aware that no training is provided in a LAS post, but training opportunities will be available in a LAT post. Supervision occurs during both LAS and LAT posts.

WHY ARE LOCUM DOCTORS NEEDED?

NHS work is continuous and there is always a need for doctors. Locum doctors are often required to fill gaps arising due to sickness, maternity leave, increased demand during a medical crisis (e.g., during the COVID-19 pandemic) and unfilled positions (new posts, retirement, resignation, and lack of appointment). A shortage of doctors can impact medical care and services in many ways (see table 1). To avoid junior doctors (JDrs) working beyond their required hours, which can have legal implications, locum doctors can be brought it to fill the gaps. Locum doctors are employed to reduce the impact of doctor shortages and to provide a smooth, uninterrupted service and maintain a high standard of quality care to patients.

Type of doctor	Location of shortage	Impact
Consultant	Ward rounds	This overall slows down the decision-making process. This results in: Patients staying longer than necessary. Patients have an increased risk of hospital-associated infection. Bed blocking so cannot admit new patients. Reduced bed side teaching of JDrs.

	Clinics	Cancellation of clinics. Increased waiting list. Patient treatment delayed. Treatment continued without adequate monitoring until next available appointment.
	On-call	Lack of senior cover leads to unsupervised JDrs. Patients not seen in a timely manner. Unnecessary admissions of patients to hospital.
	Theatre	Cancellation of surgeries. Negative effects on health, welfare and finances of patients.
Shortage of JDrs on wards	Wards	Delayed action and treatments. Overworked JDrs.
	JDrs training	JDrs are unable to attend relevant training sessions. JDrs unable to attend clinics.
	Bereavement	Delays in producing death certificates leading to extra stress for grieving friends and relatives.

Table 1: The impact of doctor shortages on patient care and training. Doctor shortages can lead to the remaining doctors being overwhelmed with conflicting tasks, like the poor doctor overleaf - something Locum doctors are sometimes used to help with.

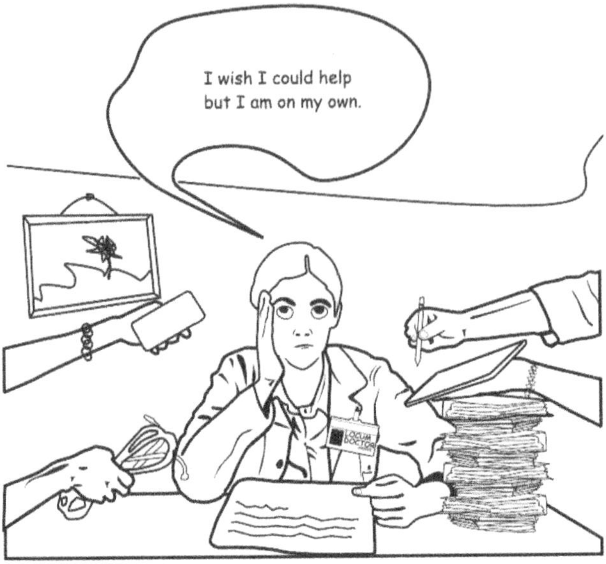

WHY DO SOME DOCTORS CHOOSE TO DO LOCUM WORK?

There are several reasons why locum work may be attractive to doctors. A short-term locum doctor may cover weekend shifts or a few weeks while another doctor is on annual leave. Long-term locum positions can be several months or longer in length. In all cases, extensions to the length of a locum position can be granted depending on the need of the trust and the quality of the work performed by the locum. Additionally, contracts can be shortened or terminated if the locum is no longer required or adequate.

Here we discuss a few examples of why doctors may take on different types of locum positions.

Occasional locum work: This is typically performed in addition to a permanent job and is usually to supplement income. For example, a trainee doctor may do occasional locum work to earn extra money to pay off their student loans. Working on-call during a weekend as a locum can be very lucrative and does not impact a permanent job.

Short-term locum work: This is often a temporary job performed while a doctor is waiting for a permanent training or consultant position.

Long-term / permanent locum work: Usually GPs, non-training grade doctors or consultants decide to be long-term or career locums. This may be because of the flexibility that locum work provides.

Last minute locum work: These positions usually arise due to last minute sick leave, a drop out or a vacancy that is unfilled. Mostly these positions cover on-call shifts and clinics or to compensate for a shortage of doctors in a specific clinical area. These posts can be filled by doctors serving in the same trust or externally.

Reasons and advantages of undertaking locum work

There are several reasons why locum work may be attractive to doctors:

- Better flexibility: Locums can choose to work part-time or full-time. They can also choose whether to work on a weekend or out of hours.
- Job location: Because there are many locum positions all around the country, it means doctors can do short-term locum work in one location and move quickly to another when they wish. This is especially important if doctors have partners that travel for their jobs. This also is attractive to doctors who want to pursue interests such as trekking or travelling alongside their work.
- Holidays: Locum work enables breaks of longer than the 2-3 weeks granted by the NHS. This is especially important for doctors with children or those who enjoy travelling.
- Extra income: Locum work allows doctors to have extra income. This can be important during natural career breaks (after foundation year 2, core training or specialist training) and prior to committing to a full-time consultant job.
- Testing future careers: Working as a locum allows doctors to experience different areas of health care and determine the specialty they wish to commit to later.

- Examination preparation: Trainee doctors can undertake locum work while preparing for exams or conducting research.

- Focused: Locum doctors can focus on specific areas of medical care e.g., clinical work, and academic or research positions.

- CV strengthening: Doctors can build their CV by working in different hospitals and in different roles. You can gain a large amount of experience and skills through different locum positions.

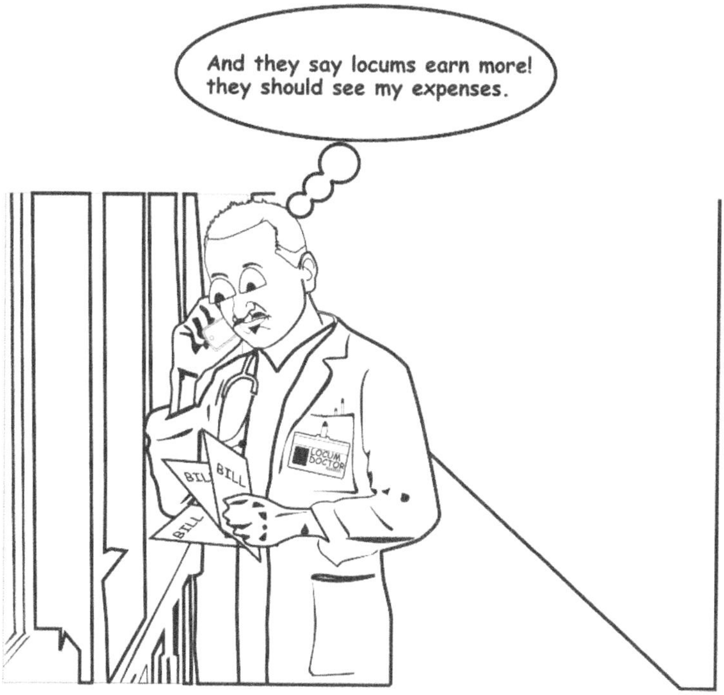

What are the disadvantages of being a locum doctor?

Despite the obvious positives of taking up a locum position, there are several disadvantages of locum work. Firstly, there are a several negative stereotypes of locums; people may assume you are not as skilled, more error prone or solely driven by money. There is a perception that doctors only take up a locum position because they are not good enough to find a substantive job. Although these assumptions are incorrect you may have to deal with unconscious bias or negative behaviour towards you as a locum doctor.

Other disadvantages of being a locum doctor include:

- Job uncertainty: There are uncertainties about when you will find a job, its location and the type of contract. These factors make future planning difficult but can be dealt with easily if you are only planning on being a locum for the short-term. However, this may be more of an issue if you are a career locum and something you need to financially prepare for.

- Job roles: Although the roles of a locum position are given during advertisement they may be vague or subject to change. You are often expected to get on with the job presented to you even though it might not be what you initially expected.

- Benefits: Unlike substantive doctors, locum doctors do not receive benefits such as paid sick or maternity leave.

- Expenses: Locum doctors incur costs for travelling and accommodation. These need to be accounted for financially.
- Learning: At each position a locum doctor will potentially have to learn a new admin and IT system, which can take time and cause delays. You will also have to quickly learn the names of your new team and how things are ran in the hospital/trust.
- Supervision roles: Locum doctors cannot participate in the supervision of junior doctors or act as an educational/clinical supervisor.
- On-call swaps: This is not as straightforward for locum doctors as it is for permanent staff members.
- Facilities: There may not be adequate office space. There may also not be permits or spaces for you to park a car.
- Missed learning opportunities: Employers can argue that since locums are paid on an hourly rate there is no obligation to provide locums with teaching or training opportunities.
- Pension: Locums experience a loss of employer pension and/or employer contribution to pension (see section on pensions).

- Pay is given weekly or fortnightly rather than monthly, which can effect budgeting. There can also be delays in receiving payments if timesheets are not submitted or signed off on time. Most agencies require a time sheet to be submitted detailing the hours worked each week by a locum. This process is as follows:

    a. Completing a detailed timesheet on a weekly basis.

    b. Completing and submitting the timesheet on time.

    c. Receiving approval from the appropriate authorising manager.

    d. Receiving approval at the level of the locum agency.

    e. Receiving and keeping track of payments (a spread sheet can help with this; an example is provided in appendix 1).

DO LOCUM DOCTORS EARN MORE THAN SUBSTANTIVE DOCTORS?

Locum doctors are paid on an hourly rate, which can be negotiated depending on your experience level. Pay is dependent on how much work is carried out and the schedule of the work e.g., weekend work pays more than weekday work. These factors can all influence the amount of pay a locum doctor receives so it could be argued that locums could receive a higher income than a substantive doctor. However, locum doctors do not receive some of the financial benefits that substantive doctors receive. Key differences in leave benefits between locum and substantive doctors can be found in table 2.

	Substantive doctor	**Locum doctor**
Annual Leave	42 days	N/A
Junior Doctor Annual Leave	32 days	N/A
Paid study leave	10 days	N/A
Professional leave	2 days/year	N/A
Career leave	Varies between trusts but typically 1-2 days/year	N/A
Funding for studies	£800-£1000	N/A
Compassionate/bereavement leave	5 days	N/A
Court hearings	As needed	N/A
Appraisal and revalidation	Free	Paid for by locum doctor
Mandatory training	Free	Paid for by locum doctor

Table 2: Key differences in leave benefits between locum and substantive doctors - this can lead to different experiences, and advantages, for both parties.

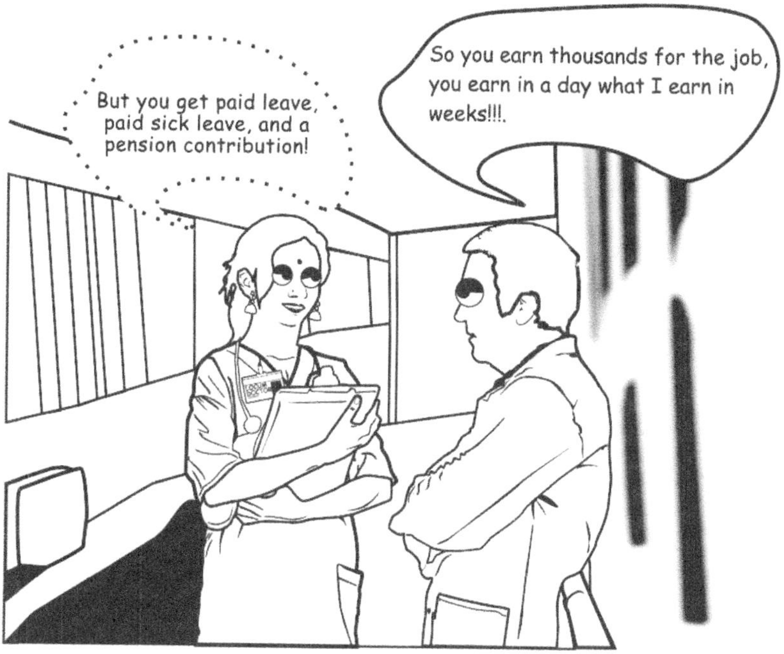

LOCUM DOCTOR PAYMENT.

Most locum doctors are employed through agencies and are paid an hourly rate, which is dependent on the grade of the position (typical values include foundation year 2: £30-75 per hour, core training doctor: £40-85 per hour and specialist trainee doctor: £50-100 per hour). Locum A&E doctors and acute medicine doctors are in particularly high demand so can negotiate a higher rate of pay more easily than other types of doctors.

Fixed term NHS trust locums are employed directly by an NHS trust and will receive a monthly salary that is on the appropriate pay scale of the substantive doctor whose work they are covering. Locums working at GPs tend to be better paid than locums employed by a hospital.

There have been several stories in the media demonstrating the large sums of money earned by some locum doctors. One story gave details of an NHS locum doctor who earned more than £500,000 a year. However, these stories rare and do not reflect the income of most locum doctors. In 2015, the NHS introduced a pay cap to discourage locums agencies charging exorbitant rates and maximum hourly rates have also been introduced for hospitals too, which can only be exceeded in exceptional circumstances. And although these rates are not set in stone, they are used as guidance for employers. These measures have been put in place to regulate the income of locum doctors.

HOW ARE LOCUM DOCTORS PAID?

When starting a locum position there are a few details you need to quickly determine so that you are paid on time. Firstly, are timesheets completed on paper or electronically? Who is required to sign your timesheets and what deadlines need to be met? It is also important to determine who is responsible for sending your timesheet to the locum agency; this could be yourself or the hospital you are working at. Retinue, STAFF flow and TempRE are examples of systems that are used by locum staff to upload timesheets online for payment directly through an NHS trust. 247Time is another system used by NHS trusts to upload locum hours worked.

There are various models of payment but the most common is pay as you earn (PAYE). Here are several preferred methods of payment for locum doctors:

PAYE: Tax is deducted at the source (your employer) depending on your tax code, which is calculated based on your annual earnings and pension contributions. Student loan repayments are also deducted from your PAYE at the source.

Limited company: This is also referred to as a personal service company. Paying locum doctors through limited companies has become less common since the implementation of off-payroll working rules (IR35). If the NHS pays through a limited company, they must do an IR35 assessment regarding the arrangement of the locum contract and will have to deduct all taxes including National Insurance (NI) before final payment is released to the limited company.

Prior to April 2017, it was the responsibility of the contractor to determine their IR35 status but now this role falls on the employer. Most NHS trusts use IR35 assessments for their locum doctors to determine the amount of tax that needs to be collected. The IR35 assessment examines the relationship between the locum doctor and the NHS trust to determine if the correct income tax and National Insurance is paid. IR35 also determines if the locum would be considered as an employee rather than a contractor if they were not using a company contract. If this is found to be the case, further tax contributions may need to be made.

Umbrella company: An umbrella company acts as the employer for locum doctors. Initially the NHS trust pays the locum agency, and they will retain a margin of this payment. The remaining money will then be transferred to an umbrella company who acts as the employer of the locum. The umbrella company will retain their margin and all employer costs. The remaining amount is then paid under PAYE. At this point expenses are also paid. Typically, locum doctors who are working through a reputable umbrella company will receive the same salary as those who are paid through the PAYE scheme.

If you work through a limited company or umbrella company it is advisable to have an accountant.

Doctors Direct: Doctors Direct is a locum service launched in 2016 that provides locum services to the NHS and is own by the Department of Health. This is an NHS professionals system and does not charge agency fees, therefore, costs and expenses are reduced and the salary of the locum is unchanged.

Direct engagement: This is an employment model that is used by many NHS trusts to allow them to make savings. A recruitment agency provides a locum doctor to an NHS trust but once employed the NHS trust will directly engage with the doctor on a fixed term basis. In this case, payment will be received directly from the NHS trust payroll allowing locum doctors to pay into an NHS pension.

There are several deductions made from a locum's salary, these are detailed below.

NI contributions as a locum doctor: NI contributions are deducted from locum pay just as they are for substantive doctors. If you are paid above the PAYE threshold employers use an employee's NI category letter to work out NI contributions. The overwhelming majority of doctors will be in category A, with the rest being category C. This is shown in table 3.

Category letter	£120 to £184 (£520 to £797 a month)	£184.01 to £967 (£797.01 to £4,189 a month)	Over £967 a week (£4,189 a month)
A	0%	12%	2%
C	0%	0%	0%

Table 3: NI contributions.

Workplace pension schemes: Workplace pension schemes were established by employers so that an employee can save money towards their retirement. There are two types of workplace pension schemes- defined benefit and defined contribution schemes, details of each can be found in table 4.

	Defined benefit scheme	**Defined contribution scheme**
Availability	Public sector worker or those in an older pension scheme.	Any employer including small businesses.
Contributions	Employee and employer contribute at time of payment.	Percentage of pay enters scheme and contributions from employer.
Amount of money accumulated	Based on your salary and amount of money contributed.	Total contribution from you and your employer plus interest.
Pension calculation at time of retirement	Based on 'final salary' or 'career average'.	The total money in the scheme at that time.
Example of pension scheme	NHS pension scheme	National Employment Savings Trust (NEST)

Nomination	Spouse or civil partner, children under the age of 23 years and in full-time education. Children who are mentally or physically impaired. Financial dependents.	Family members, friends, charity, and other organisations.

Table 4: Details of workplace pension schemes.

Private or personal pensions: In this scheme an employee must make regular contributions or a yearly lump sum into a private pension fund. Depending on your pay grade, an employer may also contribute. A private pension provider may invest the money you contribute (as a share for example) and so, the value of your pension fund may fluctuate depending on how these investments perform. Therefore, the amount you receive when you retire will be dependent on the amount of money you have paid in, how investments have performed and how you decide to receive the money e.g., regular payments or a lump sum.

Generally, 25% of your pension value is tax-free and a tax relief is paid on your pension contributions at the highest rate of income tax you pay. Therefore, basic-rate taxpayers get 20% pension tax relief whilst higher-rate taxpayers can receive 40% pension tax relief. Additional-rate taxpayers can claim 45% pension tax relief. The annual allowance for a private pension is £40,000 including contributions made by yourself, your employer, and any third-party contributions (pension tax reliefs).

WHAT ARE THE REQUIREMENTS OF A LOCUM DOCTOR?

Before you can work as a locum you must satisfy several conditions and provide relevant documentation. These are usually checked when you register at a locum recruitment agency:

- GMC registration certificates and licence to practice (for career grade doctors).
- Photographic proof of identity (passport or driving license).
- Copy of medical degree and completion of training certificate (CCT). This is essential if you are applying for GP or consultant locum positions.
- All doctors taking locum work **must** have personal professional indemnity work and show proof of their Medical Indemnity Certificate.
- Full employment history in the form of a CV.
- Contact details for a minimum of two referees, one must be an employer from the last twelve months.
- A copy of certificate verifying position on Performer's list for the relevant UK Authority if applying for a GP position.
- Valid Disclosure and Barring Service (DBS). Usually, an enhanced check is preferred.

- Valid Basic Life Support Certificate (BLS) or Adult Life Support Certificate (ALS), whichever is most appropriate.
- Immunisation records to demonstrate proof of safety to practice.
    - Dates of immunisations are required in some cases including hepatitis B (including booster). Serology evidence or vaccination record for rubella, measles, tuberculosis and personal declaration that one has had varicella infection or a serology. Recently, there are also requirements for proof of COVID-19 vaccination status.
- A recent occupational health assessment.
- Overseas doctors need a minimum of 6 months work experience in the NHS before working as a locum in the UK.

LOCUM DOCTORS AND PROFESSIONAL INDEMNITY.

It is very important for locum doctors to take out a personal professional indemnity insurance. NHS organisation insurance covers a locum doctor for complaints and negligence during employment. It does not cover criminal proceedings and GMC/disciplinary hearings. Locum doctors working in the private health care system will need to set up their own insurance.

HOW TO SEARCH FOR A LOCUM JOB.

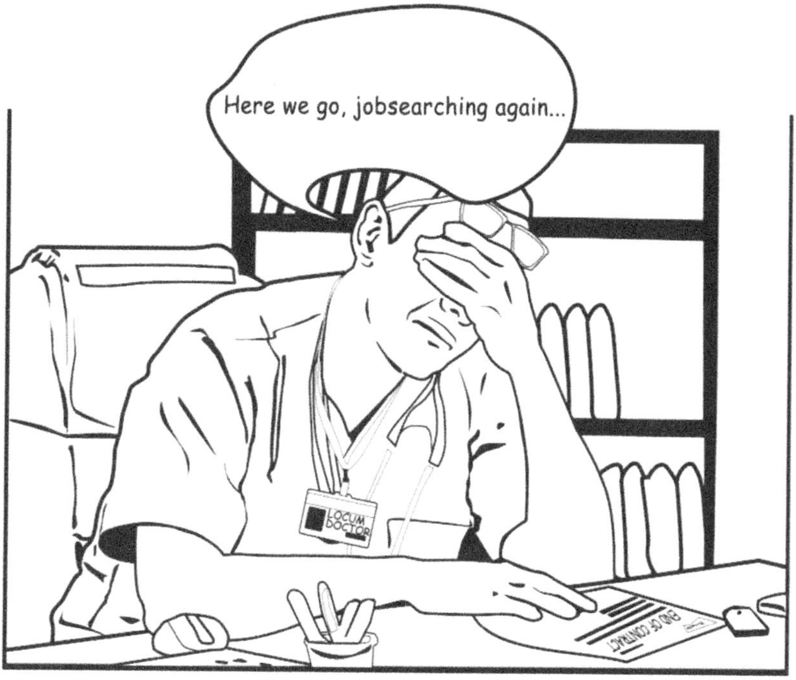

It is first important to decide whether you want to register at a locum recruitment agency or find a position directly through the NHS locum service. This will determine how you find a position and your rate of pay.

Online adverts: Many locum jobs are advertised online (NHS jobs, Indeed, BMJ websites). These tend to be fixed term contracts and payment is monthly. These positions usually cover maternity leave, sickness leave, or a vacant position.

Recruitment agencies: Locum agencies find suitable locum positions for a doctor depending on their requirements, experience, and availability. Doctors looking for locum positions typically register with multiple recruitment agencies to maximise their chances of finding a suitable job.

Direct contact: It is possible find your own locum position by contacting NHS trusts and lead consultants directly. However, this method is not that common.

HOW TO CHOOSE THE RIGHT LOCUM AGENCY.

There are many agencies specialising in locum recruitment so it is important to do research on each and find an agency that matches your preferences. Often colleagues can recommend an agency and agencies will actively advertise that they are recruiting by sending emails or attending medical conferences. Here are a few initial questions you should ask yourself before registering with a locum agency:

- How approachable is the agency?
- How responsive is the agency?
- Is the agency geographically limited? Is it regional or national?
- What is their payment procedure? Do they pay weekly or monthly?

Once you register with an agency you will be appointed a recruitment consultant/agent who will act as your point of contact at the agency and will search for suitable jobs for you. It is crucial to have a good relationship with your consultant and discuss in detail what your job preferences are. You must also tell your consultant if you have registered with several recruitment agencies and update them if you take a position.

HOW TO FIND THE RIGHT LOCUM POSITION.

Once you have decided that you want to find a locum position, you will need to find a suitable position. This is where a locum recruitment agency comes in handy. An agency will match suitable jobs with your skills, knowledge and experience. It is important to only accept jobs that you are qualified and skilled to carry out.

Before accepting a locum position it is important to ask for all details of the job and understand what is expected of you. Do not feel pressurised into accepting a role that you are not completely happy with. It is essential that you find a locum position that suits your preferences too, although this is more important if the post is long-term. Getting your first locum position will be both exciting and nerve wracking. It is important to make a good first impression as these positions are short leaving little time to impress your colleagues. It is possible that your contract could be terminated at short notice if you do not meet expectations.

CURRICULUM VITAE (CV)

A CV details your training and employment history, as well as your awards and achievements. A well-written CV should sell you to the employer and persuade them to employ you. It is crucial that your CV is up to date and tailored to the job you are applying for. Although there is not a single right way to write a CV you can find many tips online and your recruitment agency may be able to provide you with a template. An example CV is provided in appendix 2 and it is crucial that your recruitment agency always has an up to date copy of your CV.

Your CV will vary dependent on what stage of your medical career you are at since a CV reflects your training and experience. A junior doctor who recently graduated medical school will likely have a shorter CV than a senior clinical who has been working in hospitals for several years.

Although CVs vary from each individual here is an idea of information that should be included in your CV:

- Personal details (i.e., name, address and contact details)
- Qualifications (list all relevant medical degrees).
- GMC registration and date of CCT.
- Appraisal and revalidation details.

- Details of current employment including dates, location, and your role.
- Full employment history and you must account for any gaps in employment. With each role include a list of projects you have worked on/contributed to.
- Give details of research you have conducted (if appropriate).
- Give details of articles and publications you have contributed to (if appropriate).
- Relevant training courses.
- Teaching and supervisor positions held (if appropriate).
- Administrative and managerial roles held.
- Contact details of at least two referees.

AGENCY REFERRAL SCHEMES

Locum agencies earn commission and/or a fixed amount of introduction fees when they secure a job for a locum doctor in an organisation. Agencies will continually be recruiting locums and usually have referral schemes. If a registered locum doctor recommends/introduces another doctor to the agency, who later registers with the agency, they will receive a financial reward. The amount of reward varies but table 5 gives examples of incentives provided by different locum recruitment agencies.

Agency	Bonus to the doctor that makes referral (£)	Hours worked by new doctor
ID medical	200	100
Medacs	250	100
HCL Doctors	150	30
HOLT Doctors	150	30
TXM healthcare	250	100
DRC Locums	200	100
Provide medicals	350	120
Global Medics	350	120

Table 5: Examples of financial incentives for locum doctors for referrals.

PRACTICALITIES OF WORKING WITH AN AGENCY

As a locum doctor working with an agency ensure that:

- Your contact details are up to date (address, contact numbers and bank details).
- Do not accept gifts, gratuities, or money from patients or colleagues. Do not use your position for either personal or monetary gains.
- Keep your DBS updated.

- Plan your leave in advance and give sufficient notice to your employer.
- Inform both your agency contact and your line manage if you are sick or if you need to take a last-minute absence.
- Do not go to work in an inebriated condition.
- Follow local policy (infection control, complaints and mobile phone use).
- Communicate with the agency frequently.
- Maintain good record keeping especially for hours worked and payments.

HOW TO NEGOTIATE A SALARY AS A LOCUM DOCTOR

The hourly rate of a locum doctor is typically suggested by the locum agency and this is determined by availability, speciality, location, and local trust policy. A remote hospital may offer a higher rate of pay than a hospital located in a city centre. Similarly, a speciality with a shortage of doctors may offer a higher rate of pay than a speciality with an excess of doctors. Besides the hourly rate of pay, it is sometimes worth negotiating benefits such as parking, accommodation, and travel. It is important to have an open mind and be flexible when possible.

HOW TO GET STARTED IN A LOCUM POSITION

Once your position is confirmed your agency will send you your contract and reporting instructions. On your first day there will usually be the opportunity to meet the team you will be working with and get your ID card for access. If parking was not prearranged through the agency, ensure to sort this on your first day.

On your first day it is important to arrive on time to meet your colleagues, Dress smartly but appropriately. The first day will likely be spent sorting IT and admin details. Here is a list of some items that need to be addressed on your first day so that things can run as smoothly as possible:

- Receive your identity badge (remember to always wear it or have it on your person).
- Register and use your IT log in details. Your service manager/colleagues can help with this.
- Identify relevant clinical areas where you will be working and make sure you have access.
- Identify car parking and local public transport stops/stations.
- Check that you have an office or a desk space.

- Get to know the secretarial assistances and make a note of their direct line number and email addresses.
- Get details on the system used for note taking (dictaphone vs. digital recording) and letter signing (electronic or printed).
- Get details on how and where to send specialist referrals.
- Understand the on-call rota system, it is important to know what system is used for swapping duties with other members of staff.
- Give notice of any planned leave you may have. It is best to give this information before starting the job and or as soon as possible.

FIRST WEEK AS A LOCUM

After one week you should have access to the different systems used by the hospital/trust. You will probably have identified areas that you need clarification or further information, for example:

- Get clarity on multi-speciality arrangements and tertiary referrals.
- Explore departmental activities such as governance meetings, weekly teaching, multi-disciplinary team (MDT) meetings, rounds and away days.

- Explore the possibility of getting involved in an audit. This may depend on the length of your locum position.

- If multi-site working is required, check if internal travel is covered and whether a shuttle service exists for travel between sites. If it does, check departure and arrival times.

- Introduce yourself to the postgraduate centre and get details of on-going teaching activity.

DEPARTMENTAL MEETINGS AS A LOCUM

During a locum position it is likely you will not be scheduled to attend meetings. However, it is still worth finding out when these meetings are held and if you can make it based on your work schedule. While attendance at these meetings may not be required for your position, these meetings will likely be useful. Attending these meetings will help establish a better working dynamic with your colleagues and will allow you to become aware of opportunities such as teaching, supervision and audits quicker.

It is important to remember that since locum work is usually clinical and you are paid an hourly rate, some hospitals/trusts may have the understanding that you should not attend meetings within your working hours. If you are working as an NHS locum, you may be more likely to attend meetings, as you will be following the daily schedule of the substantive doctor you are covering.

TIME SHEETS

Timesheets are crucial and must be filled out correctly and on time for you to be paid. Locum doctors need to complete a timesheet to reflect the hours they have worked; this may be done directly through the hospital/trust or via your agency. It is important within your first week to identify the individual who needs to sign your timesheet. Once a timesheet has been received there is about a 2-week payment delay for weekly payrolls after the deadline has passed. If payment is directly through an agency this process may be quicker. It is important to keep a record of hours worked and receipt of payment (an example of a payment tracker can be found in appendix 1). Each time a contract ends you will receive a P45 and an annual P60. These are crucial, as you will need to submit an annual self-assessment report for HMRC to pay tax on your locum positions.

DO LOCUM DOCTORS HAVE THE SAME CLINICAL EXPERIENCE AS SUBSTANTIVE DOCTORS?

Locum doctors are employed based on their experience and skills. Typically; a panel will assess applicants' CVs to determine who has the skills required for the position. The panel will also consider references provided for each applicant. In exceptional circumstances the wrong applicant may be chosen for a position, and this is typically due to inadequate scrutiny of the CVs or a last-minute placement to maintain safety. An example of this situation is when an on-call night registrar position remains vacant. A trainee doctor may act as the locum registrar but the consultant on-call will be made aware of the situation and makes sure they are available by phone call or by staying on-site. This mitigates the immediate risk to patients and ensures the locum receives support when required.

DO LOCUM DOCTORS CONTRIBUTE TO AN ORGANISATION AND IF SO, HOW?

Locum doctors are valuable and essential members of the medical workforce and are crucial in providing on-going, uninterrupted patient care. Outside of clinical work, contributions of locum doctors vary according to the nature of their contract.

Locum contracts are relatively strict and thus, personal development is limited. This also means that in terms of work hours, locum doctors will have more hours of clinical work per week than a substantive doctor because they will not attend meetings and other commitments. Locum doctors are likely to play a crucial role following the COVID-19 pandemic, which has resulted in a backlog of patients.

Locum doctors are in a position where they can share the good and best practices of organisations where they have worked. This can be of benefit to organisations that are open to new ideas. Senior doctors who take on locum positions can bring a wealth of experience and expertise to the job and organisation.

Locum positions that are six months or longer enable locum doctors to get involved in on-going projects or to start their own project. This opportunity is not open to short-term locums. Therefore, the length of a locum contract determines how much of an impact a locum doctor can have beyond the clinical work they are employed to do.

Hospitals need medical staff that can help direct the future of the hospital, teach new doctors, and inspire other medical staff. Short-term locums may not be aware of the vision of the hospital or may have little interest since they are not taking on a permanent position. It is unlikely that a short-term locum doctor will be engaged in formal teaching and thus, will not be contributing to the training of future medical staff. Short term locums tend to 'come and go' and there is usually not enough time for them to identify a problem, work on the problem and implement a solution. There is usually no time for short-term locum doctors to engage in non-clinical work as their time is taken up by clinical work. Long-term locum positions offer greater opportunities to contribute to an organisation and leave their mark.

Table 6 outlines several reasons why locum doctors may not contribute to an organisation.

Locum doctor related	**Organisation related**
Short duration of position. Disinterest in taking on extra work. Lack of awareness about on-going projects. Lack of awareness of people to talk to about solution implementation. Lack of support from team. Worry about appearing critical.	Lack of awareness of skills of the locum. Not employing long-term locums in on-going projects. Culture related reasons. Attitudes towards locum doctors. Using locums in a service role only.

	Not providing time to develop services and participate in an audit.

Table 6: Reasons that locum doctors may not contribute to an organisation.

HOW CAN ORGANISATIONS MAKE THE MOST OUT OF A LOCUM DOCTOR?

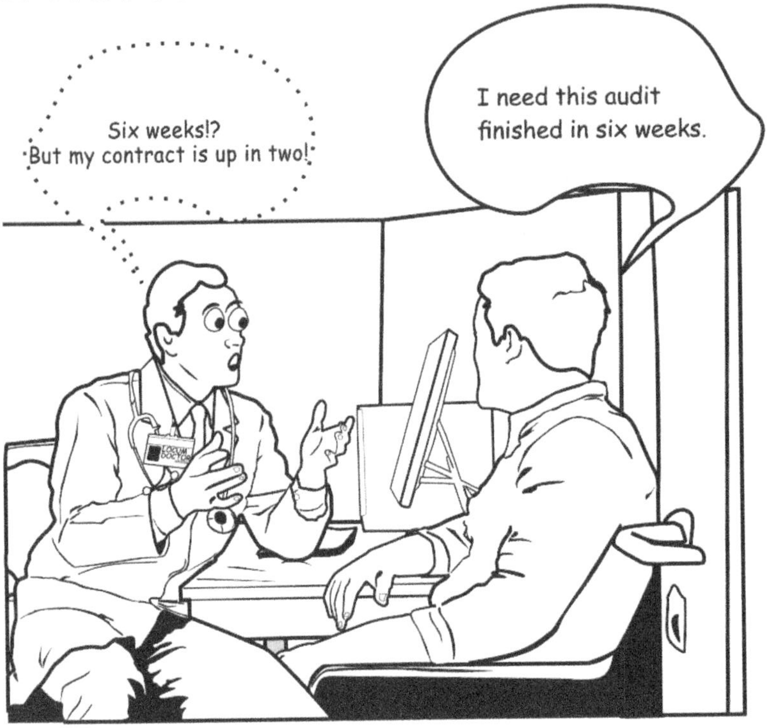

When a new member of staff joins as a locum it is important that the organisation quickly makes them comfortable and settled into the team. Examples of how organisations can do this are given below:

- Include locum doctors in group emails and messaging groups so they can become involved in activities and receive updates.

- Introduce locums to important people at the organisation: relevant consultants, those carrying out audits, postgraduate centre and education departments. It is important that locum doctors know who the research team are especially if they are staying long-term.
- Make sure locums are included in meetings if possible.
- Give details of on-call swap arrangements.
- Reassure locums that they can speak in confidence to the relevant team and can raise their concerns in a confidential manner.
- It is important to recognise the good work performed by locums, this can be done by email or in a staff meeting.
- Be sure to give updates to the locum about their contract in case of any updates and to prevent unexpected terminations.
- Ensure locums have a comprehensive introduction to IT and admin systems.
- Provide locums with a clear job plan and timetable.
- Provide locums with a safe space for their personal belongings (e.g., locker room) and an office space for admin.

- At the end of the contract, it is important that the locum is thanked for their work so that they feel a sense of appreciation. This will encourage them to take up further locum appointments.

DO LOCUM DOCTORS HAVE DIFFERENT EXPERIENCES IN DIFFERENT ORGANISATIONS?

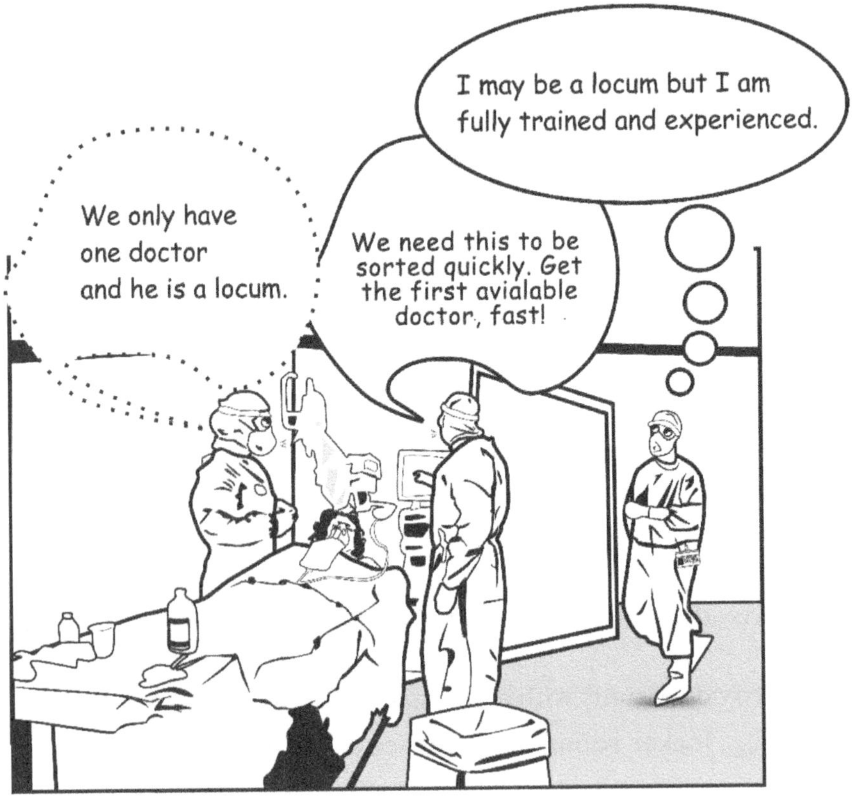

Since no two organisations are the same doctors (both locum and substantive) will have different experiences depending on the position they are hired to do and organisation they are employed by. Before starting a position, it is important to get details about the hospital/trust where you will be working.

Generally, locums will be expected to 'get on' with the job but support is there if you ask for it. However, the level of support and guidance may vary between different organisations. The longer you stay in an organisation and begin to feel like a more permanent member of the team, the more likely you will have a better experience. Therefore, your experience at an organisation may become very dependent on the length of time you are employed. A locum's experience may also differ to the experience of a substantive doctor employed by the same hospital/trust. Loyalties that hospital staff may have to permanent doctors may not be extended to locum doctors. This may be subconscious and lead to a change of behaviour or may be due to negative stereotypes and perception of locum doctors and this can lead locum doctors to feel isolated or less included.

DO LOCUM DOCTORS HAVE A CLEAR JOB PLAN?

A job plan is a weekly timetable demonstrating activities undertaken by a clinician. Tables 7 and 8 show examples of a job plan for a substantive and a locum doctor respectively. Most work carried out by locum doctors is clinical and so there is no scheduled time for managerial roles, teaching or supervision. There is also no allocated time for supporting professional activities (SPA) either. However, this may vary between employer and locum contracts. It is important to have an agreed job plan **before** agreeing to take a job and knowing your weekly schedule will make booking travel and accommodation easier.

	Mon	**Tue**	**Wed**	**Thur**	**Fri**	**Sat**	**Sun**
AM	Ward round	Clinic	SPA	Clinic	Ward round	On-call on rota	
Lunch							
PM	Admin	Clinic	Clinic	On-call	SPA		

Table 7: An example of a job plan for a substantive doctor.

	Mon	**Tue**	**Wed**	**Thur**	**Fri**	**Sat**	**Sun**
AM	Ward round/clinic					Non-working time	
Lunch							
PM	Admin	Clinic	Clinic	Clinic	Clinic		

Table 8: An example of a job plan for a locum doctor.

Although time is allocated for admin responsibilities (for both substantive and locum doctors) it is likely that some specialities will not require this time each week. This is especially the case when clinical work is mostly carried out on the ward. Admin time is more attributed to sending and processing medical results and writing discharge letters. See below examples of work that could be carried out during scheduled admin time:

- Theatre related and endoscopy: Abnormal biopsy results (post-operative) that require referral to an oncologist or a palliative care team. This also includes speaking to family members and discussing results.

- Radiology results: Abnormal radiology results showing fractures, malignancy or ruptured organs may require discussions and referrals.

- Blood tests: Abnormal blood results require communication with a GP and patients. Implementation of further investigation and action plans.

- Failed interventional procedures: This would require organisation of a follow up procedure.
- Unexpected findings: Results or findings during a procedure that were unrelated or unexpected (for example finding evidence of malignancy during a hysteroscopy) will need follow up discussions, referrals, and notes.

CAN LOCUM DOCTORS NEGOTIATE A JOB PLAN?

Once an organisation has accepted a locum doctor it is important for expectations to be outlined. This information can be found through the agency or directly from the hospital/trust. Before agreeing to a job plan it is essential for you to consider the following:

- What would be your day-to-day work schedule be?
- Would you be participating in the on-call rota? How often will you be on-call (weekdays and weekends)?
- Will you have any roles outside of clinical work?
- Is there any flexibility in the job plan?

It is important to have an open and upfront discussion before starting a locum position so that you have all the details of your contract and job plan. Be careful to check your clinic schedule and ensure that they fit within your skill set. All procedures and surgeries that fall onto a locum should be established from the beginning. It is essential that the expectations of both the locum and the hospital/trust are met and understood. When you receive your job plan make sure to mention any times or dates you may not be available but remember to be flexible.

Although it might be easier to negotiate a job plan if you are a consultant locum, there is limited scope for negotiating a job plan when you are a trainee doctor. Most of the work is allocated to you and will be based on the wards or as part of the on-call rota. Trainee doctors should identify and talk to their clinical supervisor about their work, especially when difficulties arise. There must always be someone with whom you can discuss patients and seek advice.

Table 9 shows a proposed and agreed job plan of a locum following discussions between the locum and hospital. The hospital agreed to remove the locum from the on-call rota and made alterations to both clinic and admin schedules. This left Friday free for admin work to reduce travel time and expenses.

		Mon	Tue	Wed	Thur	Fri
Proposed	AM	Supporting specialist nurses	Clinic	Admin	Clinic	Clinic
	PM	Clinic	Clinic	Clinic	Admin	On-call
Agreed	AM	Supporting specialist nurses	Clinic	Clinic	Clinic	Remote admin
	PM	Clinic	Clinic	Clinic	Clinic	Remote admin

Table 9: The proposed and agreed job plan for a locum doctor.

DO LOCUM DOCTORS NEED SUPPORTING PROFESSIONAL ACTIVITY (SPA)?

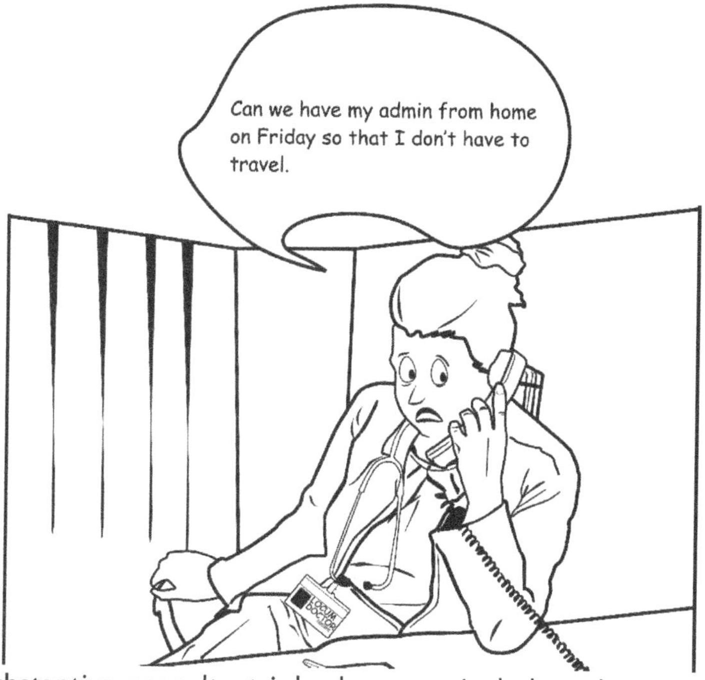

A substantive consultant job plan must include at least one SPA but most trusts allocate up to 2 or 2.5 SPA per job. On top of this there is additional professional activity (APA) that is used for teaching, training, educational activity, appraisal and revalidation, and meetings. Generally, there is no SPA entitlement for locum doctors since you are employed to provide a clinical service. Locum doctors do not have educational or supervisory roles, and therefore SPA is not usually included in their job plan. If a locum is employed through a National Health Service Professionals (NHPS) contract SPA may be allocated.

TRAVELLING AS A LOCUM DOCTOR

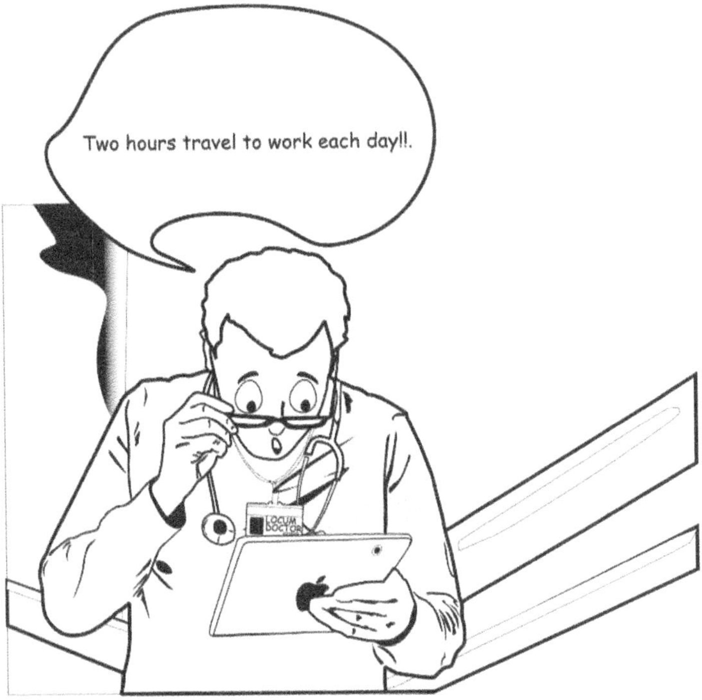

Often travel will be required for a locum position. This could be a distance that is commutable daily or may be longer and so, you may need to find accommodation close to your employer. When considering a locum position that requires travel you should consider the following:

- Total travel time.
- Start and finish time at place of work (including on-call).

- What type of travel is required (car vs. public transport) and what type of roads/lines will be taken e.g., city vs. motor way vs. countryside? These can all affect the overall commuting time and difficulty,

- Are there alternative travel routes in the event of an accident or road works?

STAYING AWAY FROM HOME

Sometimes it will not be possible to commute daily, and you will need to find accommodation to stay in. Typically, hospital accommodation is not offered and if it is, you will be charged for the room, so locum doctors typically find a hotel room to stay in if the position is short-term

Another thing to consider while staying away from home is boredom; this is especially prominent after work on an evening. Use this time to explore the local area or pursue a hobby. A downside of staying in a hotel is not being able to cook and prepare your own food, and thus, locum doctors will often spend money on takeaways or supermarket ready meals. This is not always the cheapest or most healthy option. Therefore, if possible, find accommodation that has a mini oven or a microwave.

A list of key items to bring during a stay away from home for a locum position can be found in appendix 3.

WORKING AS A LOCUM

DOES NHS INDEMNITY COVER LOCUM DOCTORS?

All doctors are legally expected to have adequate and appropriate indemnity in place from the moment they start practising medicine in the UK. This must cover the full scope of medical practice in the UK. If you work for an NHS or Health and Social Care Trust (Northern Ireland), indemnity is provided through the Clinical Negligence Scheme for Trusts (CNST), in Wales it is provided by the Welsh Risk Pool Services, in Scotland the Clinical Negligence and other Risks Indemnity Scheme provides indemnity. In Northern Ireland indemnity is provided by individual trusts and is funded by the Department of Health. This applies also for locum doctors. However, it is important to seek advice regarding the need for additional cover, which substantive doctors would get from either the Medical Protection Society or Medical Defence Union.

APPRAISAL AND REVALIDATION AS A LOCUM DOCTOR

All doctors working in the UK require GMC registration and licence. Doctors have a professional responsibility to demonstrate that they are fit to practise to ensure patient safety. This is achieved through a medical appraisal; doctors must participate in an annual appraisal and revalidation system where doctors must demonstrate that they comply with the professional standards set out in the GMC's "Good Medical Practice" Guidance. The same principles of appraisal apply to all doctors irrespective of their role or specialty. An appraisal is also an opportunity to reflect on your individual practice and performance, plan professional development and identify learning needs.

Most licensed doctors have a formal link with a designated body that provides them with an annual appraisal and supports them through revalidation, which takes place every 5 years. During revalidation a senior doctor or responsible officer (RO) within the designated body makes a recommendation every 5 years to the GMC about a doctor's fitness to practice.

Locums will be registered with an RO on a GMC site who will gather information from organisations they have worked for in the previous year, to determine if they are fit to practice. If you are working in an NHS locum post that is longer than 3 months in duration and your appraisal is due during that time, it may be possible to request an RO within the organisation you are employed. Where locum work is contracted through an agency, the agency may act as the designated body if appropriate but may charge you a fee for conducting your appraisal. If a locum is registered with several locum agencies the designated body should be the agency that secured the most contracts for the locum during the course of the appraisal year. You also have the option of finding a private appraiser, but they must be trained to conduct NHS medical appraisals and you will need to find an RO for revalidation.

The National Performers List is a list of approved substantive and locum GPs. Secondary care locums are appraised by their designated body unless they have a primary substantive post, in this case their appraisal is held by the trust where they are employed. This is also true if a locum is directly employed by the organisation on either a short or fixed-term contract. Supporting information needed for the appraisal process falls into 4 broad categories:

1. General information.

2. Keeping up to date.

3. Review of scope of practice.

4. Feedback on your practice.

There are 6 types of supporting information, which must be collected, reflected on, and discussed at the appraisal meeting:

1. Evidence of continuing professional development.

2. Quality improvement activity including an audit and case review.

3. Significant events (if any).

4. Patient feedback (once every 5 years).

5. Feedback from colleagues (once every 5 years).

6. Compliments and complaints.

As a locum doctor it can be challenging to collect all supporting information required, particularly if you have carried out several short-term positions. In particular, quality improvement activity is very difficult to obtain unless you are in a post for at least 3 months. A colleague would need to have worked with you for at least 3 months before they are able to complete a colleague feedback form. Additionally, it might be difficult to find the correct number of patients to give feedback if you have not been in a position very long. Therefore, locum doctors can focus on collecting the required information relating to the types of role they undertake rather than from every place of work. It is important to plan and if you secure a locum contract for more than 3 months you should aim to collect supporting information during that position. During your locum positions, keep note of interesting cases that you can reflect on as this can be used in the 'case reviews' portion of quality improvement activity. If you have been named in any significant events this will be communicated to you in advance. If you are named in a complaint, make sure to record all the details including your response and outcome. It is important to organise your appointment with your appraiser in advance and take feedback constructively.

The following are some pieces of information to collect during your locum position:

1. Record educational activities in a continuous professional development (CPD) diary.

2. Record internal meetings. Record dates and minutes in a separate folder. Upload an anonymised document in a CPD diary.

3. Keep feedback from teaching activities.

4. Keep a log of procedures and interesting cases you have been involved in.

5. Ensure you participate in an audit or quality improvement activity. Keep presentations and upload to an appraisal portal.

6. Collect colleague feedback.

7. Collect patient feedback.

8. Collect documents and upload them in relevant sections on time.

JUNIOR DOCTOR LOCUMS

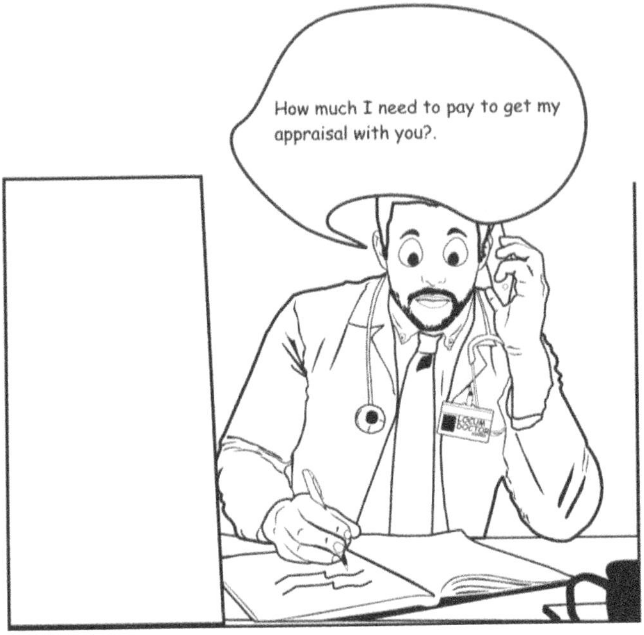

We discuss in the following section the role and responsibilities of junior doctors (JDrs) and how they can be safe and efficient locums. JDrs play a crucial role within the NHS and frequently take on extra shifts to cover gaps in the rota. Unlike consultants, JDrs do not always have a fixed or recognised job plan, and when acting as a locum they may be assigned to wards or teams to work with short notice.

JDrs are the immediate point of contact for patients, families, nurses, and ancillary staff. On a typical day JDrs are responsible for:

- The daily ward round.
- Endoscopy, theatre and/or clinics (depending on the speciality).
- Liaising with patients and family members. This includes communication of results.
- Liaising with specialist teams and social services.
- Arranging investigations for patients.
- Carrying out post-ward investigations.
- Communicating results to the relevant people.
- Prescribing and altering medications.
- Making discharge summaries.
- Participate in on-going educational activities including departmental meetings, grand round, audits and teaching other JDrs and medical students.
- Recruiting patients for research trials.
- Creating procedure lists.
- See referrals from other specialities and liaise with senior doctors (e.g., a consultant).

On-call JDrs are responsible for:

- Recording new admissions.
- Admitting and discharging patients at the emergency department.
- Reporting and seeking advice from senior clinicians.
- Carry out procedures as needed and appropriate.
- Create lists for procedures and referrals for consultants to see in ward rounds.
- Provide care to a patient admitted in their speciality (even if the patient is not in their parent team).
- Answer bleeps and participate in cardiac arrest calls.

These roles can become demanding on a JDrs for the following reasons:

- New place of work:
  - Suboptimal orientation.
  - Unaware of telephone numbers and codes, both of which take time to remember.
  - New or different policies and guidelines.
  - Getting to know a new team takes time.

- Unfamiliarity with the system:
  - IT and admin systems can vary between departments and specialities.
- Not able to participate in teaching activities.
- On-call systems can vary (bleep vs. ward based) and emergency call outs.
- On top of their clinical work JDrs will also need to fill out timesheets and payment agreements for extra shifts worked within the same organisation.

Hard-working locum JDrs will be quickly recognised by the recruiting team and senior staff. It is always important to give a good impression and the following tips may be useful for this:

- Arrive on time.
- Introduce yourself to your team.
- Provide your contact details to relevant people such as the switchboard, rota coordinator, registrar/consultant, ward nurses and fellow doctors.
- Understand department system to make coordinating work with others easier.
- Carry out your role and responsibilities with diligence and confidence.

- If a task cannot be completed, make sure you can rationalise and express your concern to a senior member of staff.
- Keep lists in safe place complying with GDPR regulations.
- Answer your bleep/phone in a timely manner.
- Make key members of staff aware of your availabilities and any absences.
- If you do need to leave your position, give notice unless in a crisis or emergency.
- Always keep track of your jobs.
- Be visible.
- Participate in on-going departmental activities.
- Be flexible and offer to help when possible and appropriate.

SAFE EXIT FROM A LOCUM POSITION

In most cases, you will know the end date of your locum position at the start of your appointment, and this should be clearly stated in your contract. In many cases, a locum contract can be extended, and this is a mutual agreement between the locum and the hospital. However, there are some instances when a contract may be terminated early, this could be because the hospital no longer requires or wants your service. Additionally, you may have found a more suitable or permanent position and wish to end your locum position early. Generally, if you have spent 6 days or less working at an organisation you need to only provide 24 hours' notice before leaving. If you have been working between 4-11 weeks' then a 2 weeks' notice period is required and if you have been working for 12 weeks or more then 4 weeks' notice is needed. In all cases written notice is required and it is important to check the exact notice period required by the hospital/trust and recruitment agency.

It is important to leave a locum position on a good note, as this will be their final impression of you. Typically, a hand over is required, especially if you have been working on-call or ward cover, so that there is a smooth transition. Make sure to specify any outstanding jobs or investigations that need to be handed over to a colleague before you leave.

If you were working in a clinic, then it is important to ensure that clinic letters are signed, results are reviews or handed over to a colleague. It is worth notifying medical secretaries when your end date is so that your letters can be signed as a priority. Also provide a list of patient investigations that are pending so that these can be followed up by another colleague. Typically, locums will leave the final afternoon of their position free of clinical work so that they can complete admin before they leave.

When leaving your position, ensure to thank your colleagues and team members, it may be a nice idea to bring a parting gift for them (such as snacks or cakes). You never know if you may wish to return to the department in future either in a locum capacity or as a permanent doctor. It is also important to thank administrative staff and secretaries who have helped you with admin work during your employment. Finally, talk to your lead consultant to see if they would be happy to provide a reference for you if you need one in the future.

UNEXPECTED ISSUES

Sickness: People get sick and are unable to go to work. As a substantive NHS doctor, statutory sick leave is included in your contract. However, this is not the case for locum doctors. Since locum doctors are paid at an hourly rate, any time off due to sickness is unpaid. This can be a huge disadvantage of locum work and for career locums. It is advised to take appropriate insurance to safeguard against this.

Mortgages and loans: The financial world sees locum work as an unstable career choice. The inconsistency and variability in working and pay can make securing a loan and mortgage difficult. The status of a locum doctor is difficult to define and can cause problems as it does not fit into standard mortgage calculators. When applying for a loan or mortgage you will have to demonstrate your annual income by providing a P60. For mortgage purposes you will need to provide a P60 and payslips for 3 years. A letter of employment will also be required, which can be difficult to obtain if you are working short-term contracts. However, it is worth asking your locum agency (if you have one) to provide an employment letter, as they may be willing to provide the necessary information.

FINANCIAL PLANNING AS A LOCUM DOCTOR

If you are planning to do locum work on a long-term basis you will need to consider how this may affect you financially in the future. It may be worth seeking help from a financial advisor who can guide you through financial planning and tailor it according to your goals. When planning for your future financially consider the following:

- Savings and investments.
- Most suitable mortgage option.
- Pension and retirement planning.

- Compliance with taxation rules and regulations.
- Life insurance, income protection and critical illness cover.

LOCUM DOCTOR REALITY CHECK

Within an organisation there may be unconscious biases towards locum doctors. The perception that locum doctors earn more money than substantive doctors is incorrect but remains. Since locums are paid on an hourly rate, organisations may wish to use them efficiently and maximise their workload. Therefore, some hospitals may give additional work to a locum that was not initially outlined in their contract. Always remember that you must be comfortable with the work you are given and both the hospital trust and the locum doctor can terminate a contract early. Negative stereotypes of locum doctors may result in you getting less respect or attention than substantive doctors, you may also feel like you do not receive the same loyalties that a substantive doctor receives. But if you continue to work hard and well with other team members then this should be overcome. One of the authors felt that she was being ignored by the senior ward staff on her first day of her job; the senior nurse communicated with the registrar and not her. But after weeks of hard work and proving herself, the situation changed, and the nurse communicated and worked well with her for the remainder of her position.

CAN LOCUM WORK BE LONG-TERM?

There are many long-term career locum doctors but this career choice is not for everybody. Many factors need to be considered before deciding to be a long-term career locum. For example, it might be important to determine if you are in a high demand speciality where there are a lot of positions you could apply to. It is also worth considering if your life and commitments are flexible, and you are willing to travel to different hospitals.

As a trainee doctor, it is not wise to do long-term locum work as this may not help advance your career. In contrast, if you intend to be a clinical fellow or a staff grade doctor then it may be suitable or appropriate to be a long-term locum.

As a GP there are many opportunities to do locum work and long-term GP locums are very common. As a more senior hospital doctor, such as a consultant, the decision of whether to do long-term locum work will depend on financial circumstances and family responsibilities.

REAL LIFE EXPERIENCES AS LOCUM DOCTOR

Consultant 1:

1. Why did you choose to be a locum?

I wanted to focus on my personal life and take time to travel the world and trek. Some of my hobbies had taken a back seat during my training period due to time and financial constraints.

2. How long have you been doing locum work?

3 years.

3. What kind of difficulties have you encountered as a locum doctor?

I experienced uncertainty in getting jobs and delays in getting paid on time. No paid leave means you must balance the number of days you take as leave during the year. The lack of sickness pay and cover means you risk losing income if you take a day off due to illness. I also experienced difficulties with tax applications, as I changed employer often it meant several different payslips and details that were missing. This also led to difficulties in securing a loan/mortgage. I also experienced some negative attitudes of colleagues, who assumed I was doing locum work for the money.

4. What have been the benefits of working as a locum doctor?

Locum work gave me more flexibility. I could control my time and days of leave to travel and trek. Since I was paid on an hourly rate, my income was better.

5. Have you considered switching back to a substantive post?

Yes, I plan to switch in the future.

6. Is locum work financially rewarding?

Yes.

7. Have you come across a situation where you had to leave an agreed job?

Not yet.

8. Would you recommend being a long-term locum to your registrar?

No, not long-term as the uncertainties of finding a suitable job close to your home is stressful. You may have to work far from home and see your family only on weekends. Also, you may not be able to develop other skills like leadership, management, and teaching, which are important as a consultant.

9. What is the longest period you have gone without working and was this? If not, did you worry about how you would cope financially?

It was about two months, several years ago now. It was not intentional, but a product of new financial measures being introduced by the local trust. When it became clear that this wasn't going to be resolved quickly, I moved my base of operations and found work again quickly. I did worry about my long-term prospects, if this were to become a nationwide issue, but I had made sure to accumulate some savings so that I wasn't in immediate jeopardy, and it became apparent that I could readily find work by moving further North.

10. Do you miss anything about being a substantive doctor, if so, what?

Yes, the certainty of a secure job closer to family and home with a stable monthly income and a pension.

Consultant 2:

1. Why did you choose to be a locum?

It was not a choice, it was the only option for me at the time because there was no permanent training available. I was a graduate from my home country, where I had already reached consultant level. To start from the beginning in NHS was for me a waste of time. I discussed my situation with one of the Deanery's in London at the time and they acknowledged that it would be unfair for me to start from the beginning given my previous experience. I applied for 2 or 3 specialist registrar jobs without success. It was very difficult at that time as it was very competitive. I decided it was a good idea to work as a locum, consolidate everything and try to tick the boxes. My first job in the UK was as a registrar clinical research fellow in a London hospital. After 2 years I then went to study for further degrees. I then started to work to support myself financially. So, my two reasons for working as a locum were to support myself financially and to get experience of working in the NHS.

2. How long have you been doing Locum work?

   I have worked as a locum since 2005.

3. What kind of difficulties have you encountered as a locum doctor?

   We have lots of difficulties. One is the fact that as a locum you change hospitals frequently. This is very challenging because each trust will be run differently so you need to quickly learn and adapt. The methods of communication used by each trust will also vary. This is extremely challenging if you are a foreigner and you enter a semi-senior level in the NHS. When working with a new team, you have limited knowledge of the team and working environment. The attitude and support of hospitals varies, some individuals are friendly while others have an attitude of 'they are a locum, they are not qualified or know anything' so they may treat you worse than a substantive doctor.

Colleagues may also place more pressure on you to work much harder than they would expect from a substantive doctor. Often it feels like you must prove your abilities. Changing environments can be challenging, as you do not know what to expect from other people or their attitudes towards locum doctors.

Another challenge is how to limit abuse. Because you are a locum some organisations may try to give you the "donkey-work" and give you a hard time. To overcome this you need to believe in yourself and have confidence in your professional abilities. You must also be of the mind-set that your work is for your patients rather than for the hospital/trust. When you work in this way and see the appreciation from patients that is a major reward.

4. What have been the benefits of working as a locum?

I cannot deny that before 2017 locum work did have its financial benefits, but after introducing IR35 I personally feel that these benefits no longer exist. The main benefit now of locum work is its flexibility, if you do not like working in a hospital then you only need to give a few weeks' notice and you can leave to find another position. You can also decide when to take your holiday leave without planning a year in advance. This works well for me. Even when I was in my home country I worked as an independent consultant, so I am not used to the idea of planning far ahead for my leave or planning around others.

5. Have you considered becoming a substantive doctor?

I have been fortunate in that wherever I have worked I have always been offered a substantive position. I used to work in a prominent teaching hospital in London from 2007 to 2010. The Medical Director, CEO, and operations manager tried to persuade me to stay by offering me 13 PA. I declined because my original intention had been to return to my home country after securing my UK qualifications. Unfortunately, after 2011 there were a lot of problems in my country so I was not able to return. We kept hoping the situation would improve but it did not. So, I have stayed in the UK as a locum doctor, I prefer the flexibility and slightly better income, so I am not interested in a substantive position.

6. Have you come across a situation where you had to leave an agreed locum job early?

Yes, I worked in a very disorganised hospital where the trust was led by a business manager rather than a clinician. I felt there were systemic and management failures, which negatively impacted on the quality of patient care and this led to problems that were not due to the doctors. I was not happy and the situation made my life difficult. My contract was for 6 months, but I only stayed for 2 weeks and I gave in my notice and left.

7. Would you recommend long-term locum work to your registrar?

   This very much depends on the registrar and what they want in their medical career. Indeed, if you were young (30-35 years) I would not advise it but if you are 40-45 years then maybe it is a good career option. If you want to enter an academic career, then locum work is not a good option. Whether you decide to be a short-term or long-term locum really depends on what you value and what you want in your medical career.

8. What is the longest period you have gone without working? Was it intentional? Did you worry about how you would cope financially during this time?

   In 2005, one of my friends who at the time was in the same situation as me stated that I was mad to be doing locum work, and that it is only for stupid people. But, as a locum I can work when I want, it is flexible and allows me to take holidays when I want to. There is not an option for me not to work, because hospital trusts will call me directly and through my agency to discuss a locum contract, so I have not had to go a period without work.

9. Do you miss anything about being a substantive doctor? And if so, what?

   I envy substantive consultants because they can take sickness and holiday leave and still get paid whereas I cannot.

Consultant 3:

1. Can you explain how you became a career locum?

   It was quite a big decision at the time as I had been a consultant for nearly 20 years. However, my job at the time was not the job I had hoped for, especially in terms of pressure and responsibility. There was a huge on-call commitment. So, I just felt this was the time for me to try something different. It was a big step and a huge change, and to be honest most people probably thought that I was crazy. It has now been over 5 years and I have never regretted my decision to become a long-term locum.

2. What were your concerns at the time?

   The biggest worry I had was wondering if I would get a job. But I think we are quite fortunate in medicine that there are many options for jobs. My other major concern was whether I could get a job close to home. My first locum job was in Nottinghamshire, and I lived away from home during the week.

3. Did the thought occur to you that you would be doing several of short-term jobs?

   Most of my jobs have been a minimum of 4 months and my longest job was nearly 3 years. At the end of the day though, sometimes you must go with what is available even if this means taking on short-term positions. If you do not then you have to make sure you have a financial buffer to support yourself if you decide to wait for a more appropriate job to become available.

4. Do you think it is the case that locum work attracts people who want to pursue other interests and hobbies?

   Definitely, and that is why locum work suits some people's lifestyle. A key reason why many people become a locum is that it is flexible and allows doctors more easily to pursue hobbies and interests outside of work.

5. What kind of problems did you encounter in your first few weeks as a locum?

   The biggest problems I faced when starting a new locum position was meeting new teams constantly. I think some of the other problems I faced are more administrative; IT is a major headache. Also, a practical issue is finding appropriate places to store your belongings, you might not necessarily have an office or desk space so sorting this can sometimes take time.

6. Have you ever considered going back to a substantive job?

   Interestingly, it was only recently that I thought I would be a locum for a long time. Although, I anticipate towards the end of my career I might go back to substantive work; mostly because of the pension it would give me. Because of the nature of my job, I encounter many sick people and it has made me wonder what would happen if I became ill and needed to take time off work unpaid. So, I think if the right permanent job appeared at the right time, I would go for it. It is something I would consider but I am not keen on working full-time anymore or being on-call.

7. If your registrar came to you and said that they wanted to be a career locum, what would be your response?

   At this stage of their career I would not encourage it. At the age of 30 I think it is too young to become a career locum, it is too risky. This is especially the case if you have a young family; it is not convenient for you to be travelling to different locum positions. So overall, I think it depends on your career aspirations and your personal circumstances. I know a lot of registrars will take on locum jobs initially because they are not sure what they want, or they need extra money for mortgages etc. But they also need to decide if they want to be a locum long-term.

8. Are there any other points that you would like to raise?

   Firstly, it is really important to plan ahead before an appraisal, as this can be difficult for doctors doing several short-term locum positions. If you find yourself in the position of doing a 6-month or longer locum post, this is a good opportunity to get appraisals (such as patient and colleague feedback) because you cannot get this information during a shorter contract. Another problem I encountered was applying for mortgages, so this is something you need to be aware of as I learnt this too late. If you are a locum doctor you are perceived as not having a stable or secure job. Therefore, it is risky for lenders to give you loans or mortgages.

9. Is it good to find locum positions directly through the NHS or is it better to find positions through an agency?

That is a brilliant question. I have never worked as an NHS locum simply because the rates of pay are quite different to other locum positions. However, there are some benefits in the NHS locum system. For example, if you work as an NHS locum you can still contribute to your NHS pension, which is important. Secondly, you are more likely to get a longer contract with an NHS locum position. So obviously that is attractive as it means you do not have to move around as much. I think you also receive some other benefits such as some paid sickness, study, and annual leave just not as much as substantive doctors.

Thank you

I hope you have found this book useful. Please email ranjnagargapril-book@yahoo.com to provide any feedback or anything else you would like included in the subsequent editions of this book.

APPENDICES

APPENDIX 1: AN EXAMPLE OF PAYMENT TRACKER.

Hospital	Role	Week commencing	Hours worked	Rate/hour	Submitted?	Received?
A	Consultant	04/01/2022	42	100	Yes	4200
A	Consultant	11/01/2022	36	100	No	No

APPENDIX 2: AN EXAMPLE CV.

Personal details

Name:

Address:

Email:

Telephone number:

General Medical Council number

Qualifications:

MBBS year

MRCP/MRCS or similar (UK) year

CCT (speciality) year

Current appointment

Start date and end date

Locum consultant speciality:

Hospital name/NHS trust:

Responsibilities (examples):

- Management of in-patients and clinic.

- GIM ward.
- Junior doctor supervision and teaching.
- List of clinics/procedures/theatres attended.
- On-call commitments.

Previous role responsibilities

Clinical:

- Management of theatre flow and waiting list initiative.
- Established new service: if relevant give an example.

Management:

- Leading quality improvement project in XX speciality. Show financial impact if possible or benefits provided.
- Quality improvement project. Give an example, this could be related to infection control.
- Developing pathways for new admissions if relevant.
- Supervision of junior doctors/medical students.

Academic:

- Give details of awards won.
- Details of regular teaching commitments of medical students etc.
- Organisation and teaching of medical courses.
- Examiner role.

- Role of providing updates within trust/hospital and between hospitals/trusts.

Here you may also include other roles or personal achievements that you may have if they are relevant to the position.

Publications

Details of involvement in articles published in peer reviewed journals.

Previous appointments

August 2016 to January 2021: Full time substantive consultant surgeon (insert details of location).

March 2016 to July 2017: Locum consultant surgeon (maternity cover, insert details of location).

November 2015 to March 2016: Locum consultant surgeon (insert details of location)

August 2009 to October 2015: Specialist register (rotation, insert details of location)

References

Give details of individuals who can provide references (name, email, and telephone numbers).

SHO/CMT APPOINTMENTS IN GENERAL / INTERNAL MEDICINE

George Eliot Hospital, City	Dec 2008 to July 2009
XXX District General Hospital	Feb 2007 to Dec 2008

Foundation year training: List deanery/hospital/dates

PUBLICATION: Insert list in chronological order (most recent first)

Published Abstract/Presentations

- Insert list in chronological order (most recent first)
- Highlight light any awards
- Distinguish between oral, poster and abstract only

Interests: Insert anything that you do and enjoy in free time (gardening, photography, hiking adventures): be prepared to talk about them in your interview

"One of the authors with Scuba diving as a hobby ended up having a conversation with a panel member on hyperbaric oxygen during interview (She got the job)"

Communication Skill/Languages: Insert what is your unique selling point: think: excellent teacher, great team worker, multilinguistic, knowledge of the law, skilled in finances etc.

Personal attributes

REFERENCES: Dr xxxx, Clinical director XXX, insert hospital name and contact details

APPENDIX 3: LIST OF ITEMS TO TAKE WHEN TRAVELLING FOR A LOCUM POSITION.

1. Clothing:

    a. Daily wear, work wear, warm clothes, jacket, nightwear, socks, and underwear.

    b. Bedding: bed spread/cover, duvet cover (with or without duvet) if not provided by accommodation.

    c. Shoes: Comfortable work shoes, walking shoes and slippers.

2. Utensils: (unless provided in accommodation)

    a. Kettle and mugs.

    b. Plates, bowls and utensils.

    c. Cooking pots and pans.

3. Tea, coffee, and snacks. Dietary related items.

4. Electronics:

    a. Mobile phone, laptop, iPad, kindle, and chargers.

    b. Hair dryer.

    c. Shaver.

    d. Beard trimmer.

5. Toiletries:
    a. Towels.
    b. Soap and hand sanitizer.
    c. Toothbrush and toothpaste.
6. Writing materials and books.
7. Hobby related items e.g., camera.
8. Miscellaneous (if and as needed):
    a. Contact lens solution and storage container.
    b. Spectacles and sunglasses.
    c. Personal first aid kit and medication.

LINKS

https://improvement.nhs.uk/documents/309/Reducing_reliance_on_medical_locums_-_a_practical_guide_for_medical_directors.pdf

https://www.ihpo.manchester.ac.uk/research/projects/the-use-of-locum-doctors-in-the-nhs/

https://www.england.nhs.uk/medical-revalidation/doctors/locum-ad/

https://www.nhsprofessionals.nhs.uk/DoctorsDirect

https://www.gmc-uk.org/-/media/documents/what-our-data-tells-us-about-locum-doctors_pdf-74371150.pdf

GMC tool to find connection for revalidation

https://www.gmc-uk.org/registration-and-licensing/managing-your-registration/revalidation/my-db-tool

https://www.whatthebleep.co.uk/locumagencybonus?gclid=Cj0KCQiA5vbBRCRARIsAJBKc6KMVhu5jrWZvER3VJkxnTbCwHYw_BbVoTgJsnmlHr939qY7AeXfBQgaAvb_EALw_wcB

https://www.medacs.com/doctor/locum-doctor-your-guide-to-becoming-a-locum-doctor

ABBREVIATIONS

CPD: Continuous professional development

CV: Curriculum Vitae

GMC: General Medical Council

GPs: General practitioners

JDrs: Junior doctors

MDT: multi-disciplinary team

NHS: National Health Service

SPA: Supporting professional activity

ABOUT US

We currently publish over 110 titles across a range of subject areas – covering specialised admissions tests, examination techniques, personal statement guides, plus everything else you need to improve your chances of getting on to competitive courses such as medicine and law, as well as into universities such as Oxford and Cambridge.

Outside of publishing we also operate a highly successful tuition division, called UniAdmissions. This company was founded in 2013 by Dr Rohan Agarwal and Dr David Salt, both Cambridge Medical graduates with several years of tutoring experience. Since then, every year, hundreds of applicants and schools work with us on our programmes. Through the programmes we offer, we deliver expert tuition, exclusive course places, online courses, best-selling textbooks and much more.

With a team of over 1,000 Oxbridge tutors and a proven track record, UniAdmissions have quickly become the UK's number one admissions company.

Visit and engage with us at:

Website (UniAdmissions): www.uniadmissions.co.uk

Facebook: www.facebook.com/uniadmissionsuk

YOUR FREE BOOK

Thanks for purchasing this Ultimate Book. Readers like you have the power to make or break a book –hopefully you found this one useful and informative. *The Oxbridge Medical Society* would love to hear about your experiences with this book. As thanks for your time we'll send you another ebook from our Ultimate Guide series absolutely FREE!

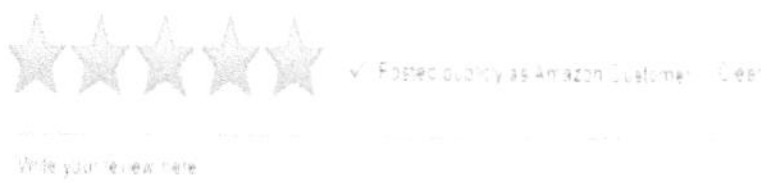

How to Redeem Your Free Ebook

1) Find the book you have on your Amazon purchase history or your email receipt to help find the book on Amazon.

2) On the product page at the Customer Reviews area, click 'Write a customer review'. Write your review and post it! Copy the review page or take a screen shot of the review you have left.

3) Head over to www.uniadmissions.co.uk/oxbridge-free-book and select your chosen free ebook!

Your ebook will then be emailed to you – it's as simple as that!

Printed and bound by CPI Group (UK) Ltd, Croydon, CR0 4YY
02/11/2026
02243551-0001